CIALIS

**Basic Guide On How To Boost Libido, Get Hard
,Stay Healthy , Stay Active Using Cialis**

Dr. J. Christorph

Table of Contents

Chapter1

Introduction to cialis

Cialis, also known by its generic name tadalafil, is a medication used to treat erectile dysfunction (ED) and benign prostatic hyperplasia (BPH). It belongs to a class of drugs called phosphodiesterase-5 (PDE5) inhibitors, which work by relaxing the muscles and increasing blood flow to certain areas of the body. Cialis was first approved by the US Food and Drug Administration (FDA) in 2003, and since then has become a popular and effective treatment for ED. It is manufactured by the pharmaceutical company Eli Lilly and is available in various doses, ranging from 2.5 mg to 20 mg. Erectile dysfunction is a common condition that affects millions of men worldwide. It is characterized by the inability to get or maintain an erection, which can greatly impact a man's sexual performance and overall well-being. While ED can be caused by various factors such as stress, anxiety, and underlying health conditions, it is mostly attributed to reduced blood flow to the penis. This reduced blood flow can be caused by factors such as smoking, high blood pressure, and diabetes. Cialis works by blocking the action of the enzyme PDE5, which breaks down nitric oxide in the body. Nitric oxide is a chemical that helps to relax the muscles in the penis, allowing for increased blood flow and ultimately, an erection. By inhibiting PDE5, Cialis helps to maintain the levels of nitric oxide in the body, resulting in improved blood flow to the penis and prolonged erections. One of the key advantages of Cialis is its long-lasting effects. While other ED medications such as Viagra only last for 4-6 hours, the effects of Cialis can last for up to 36 hours. This makes it a popular choice for those looking for a longer-lasting solution for their erectile dysfunction. In addition to treating erectile dysfunction, Cialis is also prescribed for the treatment of benign prostatic hyperplasia (BPH). BPH is a condition where the prostate gland becomes enlarged, causing difficulty with urination. Cialis works by relaxing the muscles in the prostate and bladder, which helps to ease the symptoms of

BPH. When taking Cialis, it is important to follow the recommended dosage and usage instructions provided by your doctor. It is typically taken once a day, either with or without food. The effects of Cialis can be felt within 30 minutes of consumption and may last up to 36 hours. It is important to note that Cialis does not cause an automatic erection, but rather requires sexual stimulation to work. Cialis comes in the form of tablets, which should be taken whole and not crushed or chewed. It is not recommended to take more than one tablet in a 24-hour period. Overdosing on Cialis can increase the risk of side effects, such as headache, dizziness, nausea, and priapism (a painful erection lasting more than four hours). Like any medication, Cialis may cause side effects in some individuals. The most common side effects reported include headache, facial flushing, upset stomach, back pain, and muscle aches. These side effects are usually mild and subside within a few hours. However, if these side effects persist or become severe, it is important to seek medical attention. It is important to note that Cialis should not be taken with certain medications, particularly those containing nitrates, as this can cause a dangerous drop in blood pressure. It is also not recommended to take Cialis if you have a history of heart disease, stroke, or low blood pressure. It is always best to consult with a healthcare professional before starting any new medication. In conclusion,

Cialis is a widely-used and effective medication for the treatment of erectile dysfunction and benign prostatic hyperplasia. Its long-lasting effects and fewer side effects compared to other ED medications make it a popular choice among men. With the guidance of a healthcare professional and following the recommended dosage, Cialis can help improve the quality of life for those struggling with ED and BPH

Chapter2

Uses of cialis

1. Erectile Dysfunction (ED) Erectile dysfunction is a condition where a man is unable to achieve or maintain an erection sufficient for sexual intercourse. It is a common male sexual problem that affects men of all ages. Cialis works by increasing blood flow to the penis, which helps to achieve and maintain an erection. It is one of the most effective medications for ED, with studies showing that it can significantly improve erectile function in men. 2. Benign Prostatic Hyperplasia (BPH) Benign prostatic hyperplasia is a non-cancerous enlargement of the prostate gland that can cause urinary symptoms

such as a weak urine stream, frequent urination, and urinary urgency. Cialis is FDA approved for the treatment of BPH, and studies have shown that it can improve urinary flow and reduce urinary symptoms in men with BPH. It works by relaxing the muscles in the prostate and bladder, which can help to improve urine flow. 3. Pulmonary Arterial Hypertension (PAH) Pulmonary arterial hypertension is a rare, but serious condition where the blood pressure in the arteries leading to the lungs is too high. This puts a strain on the heart and can lead to heart failure. Cialis has been approved for the treatment of PAH, and studies have shown that it can improve exercise capacity and delay the progression of the disease. It works by relaxing the blood vessels in the lungs, which helps to reduce the strain on the heart. 4. Raynaud's Phenomenon Raynaud's phenomenon is a condition where the blood vessels in the fingers and toes constrict in response to cold temperatures or stress, leading to decreased blood flow and numbness, tingling, and pain in the affected area. Cialis has been found to improve symptoms in patients with Raynaud's phenomenon by relaxing the blood vessels and increasing blood flow to the affected areas. 5. High Altitude Pulmonary Edema (HAPE) High altitude pulmonary edema is a condition where fluid accumulates in the lungs at high altitudes, leading to shortness of breath, coughing, and fatigue. It is a potentially life-threatening condition that can occur in high-altitude climbers or individuals quickly ascending to high altitudes. Studies have shown that Cialis can prevent the onset of HAPE by increasing blood flow to the lungs and reducing the strain on the heart. 6. Female Sexual Dysfunction Cialis has also been found to be effective in treating female sexual dysfunction, especially in women who have not responded to other treatments. This includes conditions such as female sexual arousal disorder and hypoactive sexual desire disorder. Studies have shown that Cialis can increase blood flow to the genital area in women, leading to improved sexual function and satisfaction. 7. Antidepressant-Induced

Sexual Dysfunction Antidepressants are often prescribed to treat depression, but they can also cause sexual side effects, such as decreased libido, erectile dysfunction, and anorgasmia. Cialis has been found to be effective in improving sexual function in men and women who are experiencing sexual side effects from antidepressants. It works by increasing blood flow to the genital area, which can counteract the sexual side effects of antidepressants. 8. Chronic Pelvic Pain Syndrome (CPPS) Chronic pelvic pain syndrome is a condition that causes pain and discomfort in the pelvic area. It can be caused by a variety of factors, including inflammation, nerve damage, and psychological factors. Studies have shown that Cialis can improve symptoms in men with CPPS by relaxing the pelvic muscles and increasing blood flow to the affected area. 9. Infertility In some cases, ED may be a symptom of an underlying medical condition, such as low testosterone, which can also affect sperm quality and fertility. Cialis has been found to improve sperm quality and increase fertility in men with ED. It works by increasing blood flow to the testes, which can improve testosterone production and sperm quality. 10. Bodybuilding and Athletic Performance Enhancement Some athletes and bodybuilders use Cialis as a performance-enhancing drug because it can increase blood flow and oxygen delivery to the muscles, leading to improved endurance and strength.

However, this use is not supported by scientific evidence, and Cialis is not approved for this purpose.

C hapter2

Dosage of cialis

The recommended starting dose of Cialis for most patients is 10mg, taken before sexual activity. It is important to note that Cialis does not cure ED, but instead helps to temporarily increase blood flow to the penis, allowing for an erection to occur with sexual stimulation. As such, it is recommended that it be taken as needed, rather than on a daily basis, and not more than once within a 24-hour period. For those with more severe cases of ED, a higher dosage of 20mg may be prescribed. Similarly, for those with BPH, the dosage may be increased to 5mg once daily. However, it is important to follow the instructions of a healthcare provider and never exceed the recommended dosage without consulting a doctor. Factors Affecting Dosage The dosage of Cialis may vary depending on several factors such as age, medical history, and other medications being taken. For instance, those over the age of 65 may need a lower dosage due to the body's decreased ability to clear the drug. Similarly, those with liver or kidney impairments may require a lower dosage as these organs are responsible for metabolizing and excreting the drug. Patients taking certain medications, such as nitrates for chest pain, should not take Cialis as it can cause a dangerous drop in blood pressure. Importance of Consulting a Healthcare

Provider It is crucial to consult a healthcare provider before starting any dosage of Cialis. This is because they are trained to assess an individual's medical history and current health condition to determine the appropriate dosage. They may also recommend certain lifestyle changes or other treatments that could improve the effectiveness of Cialis. It is also essential to inform the healthcare provider of any other medications being taken, as they may interact with Cialis and increase the risk of side effects. Additionally, if an individual has a history of heart disease, stroke, or low blood pressure, they should inform their doctor before taking Cialis. Dosage Adjustments In certain cases, a healthcare provider may adjust the dosage of Cialis depending on an individual's response to the medication. If the recommended dose is not effective or well-tolerated, they may increase or decrease it accordingly. Some individuals may also find that a lower dosage is enough to achieve the desired results, while others may need a higher dosage. This is why it is essential to work closely with a healthcare provider and report any side effects or lack of effectiveness experienced while taking Cialis. It is also important to note that the effects of Cialis may vary from person to person. While some may experience an improvement in their erectile function with the recommended dosage, others may not. In such cases, a healthcare provider may consider alternative treatment options or adjust the dosage accordingly. Possible Side Effects Like any medication, Cialis has potential side effects, although they are usually mild and do not require medical attention. The most commonly reported side effects include headache, flushing, indigestion, back pain, and muscle aches. These side effects typically subside within a few hours and can be managed with over-the-counter pain medication. More severe side effects, such as vision or hearing changes, chest pain, and an allergic reaction, are rare but should be reported to a healthcare provider immediately. In the event of a prolonged, painful erection lasting more than four hours, medical attention should be sought to avoid permanent damage to the penis.

Chapter3

Side effects of cialis

The most common side effects of Cialis include headache, flushing, upset stomach, back pain, muscle aches, stuffy or runny nose, and pain in the arms or legs. These side effects are usually mild, and they usually improve with continued use of the medication. If any of these side effects persist or become bothersome, it is important to consult a doctor. Headaches – Headaches are the most commonly reported side effect of Cialis. They typically occur within an hour of taking the medication and can last up to 48 hours. To manage headaches, doctors may recommend over-the-counter pain relievers or lowering the dosage of Cialis. Flushing – Flushing is another common side effect of Cialis and is characterized by a redness of the face or body. This is caused by the dilation of blood vessels due to the increased blood flow caused by the medication. Flushing is usually mild and resolves on its own, but if it is bothersome, drinking plenty of water and staying cool can help. Upset Stomach – Some people may experience an upset stomach after taking Cialis. This can manifest as indigestion, bloating, or nausea. To prevent this, it is recommended to take the medication with food. If symptoms persist, doctors may prescribe medications or suggest lifestyle changes to manage stomach upset. Back Pain and Muscle Aches –

Back pain and muscle aches are reported by some individuals taking Cialis. These side effects are usually mild and resolve with time. However, if the pain is severe or persists, it is important to consult a doctor. Serious Side Effects to Watch Out For: While rare, there are some serious side effects of Cialis that require immediate medical attention. These include: - Priapism – This is a prolonged and painful erection that lasts for more than four hours. It is a medical emergency that can cause damage to the tissue of the penis if not treated promptly. If you experience an erection that does not go away after four hours, seek medical help immediately. - Changes in Vision or Hearing – Cialis can cause changes in vision such as blurred vision or decreased vision. It can also cause ringing in the ears or sudden hearing loss. If you experience any of these symptoms while taking Cialis, stop taking the medication and seek medical attention. - Allergic Reactions – Some individuals may experience allergic reactions to Cialis. Symptoms may include difficulty breathing, rash, itching, or swelling of the face and tongue. If you experience any of these symptoms, seek immediate medical attention. Interactions with Other Medications: Cialis may interact with some medications, causing potential side effects. It is important to inform your doctor about all the medications you are taking, including prescription drugs, over-the-counter medications, vitamins, and supplements to avoid potential interactions. Some medications that may interact with Cialis include: - Nitrates – Cialis should not be taken with medications containing nitrates, as it can cause a sudden drop in blood pressure, which can be dangerous. - Alpha-Blockers – These are used to treat high blood pressure and benign prostatic hyperplasia (BPH). Taking them with Cialis can also cause a sudden drop in blood pressure. - Other ED Medications – Taking Cialis with other ED medications can lead to an overdose and severe side effects. - Antibiotics and Antifungals – These may increase the levels of Cialis in the body, leading to potential side effects. How to Minimize

Side Effects: To minimize the occurrence of side effects, always take Cialis as prescribed by your doctor. Do not take more than the recommended dose or use it more frequently than recommended. Taking it on an empty stomach can increase the absorption of the medication, leading to more severe side effects. Avoid alcohol and grapefruit while taking Cialis, as they may increase the risk of side effects. If you experience any side effects of Cialis, it is important to discuss them with your doctor. They may adjust the dosage or prescribe a different medication to manage your symptoms. In most cases, the benefits of Cialis for treating ED and enlarged prostate symptoms outweigh the potential side effects. However, it is crucial to be aware of them and take necessary precautions to minimize their impact.

The end

Made in the USA
Las Vegas, NV
14 May 2024